Dessert First Diet

Conquer and Cure your Cravings…
…before they Blossom into Binges

Diet Smarter, not Harder

Written by:
Brian Shell

2

Table of Contents:

Dedication to my Mom

This book is dedicated to my mother. I love you Mom!

Also, I dedicate this book to _Foxy Roxy the Feral Fat Cat_ who adopted me as her owner after my dog passed away in 2008... because simply, this food philosophy worked on her as well. So if the "_spoonful of sugar to help the medicine go down_" methodology can work for a cat, it can help you.

Now though, I can't call her that anymore. She's lost weight.

Now... she's "_Roxy – the Lean Mean Feline Machine._"

She likes it when I tell her she's lost weight too.

Somehow she _knows_ and acknowledges it.

My food theory worked on us both.

I hope it will help you as well.

Just put it into practice.

Acknowledgements

Wow… Since publishing my first book in December of 2009 and seeing myself on TV to promote it, quite a transformation has occurred within me.

It's funny how they say that being on TV adds 10 pounds… but the reality is that if you truly feel you need to lose weight, do it. Don't talk the talk if you aren't going to walk the walk. Put it into everyday practice so your choices become healthy habits for life. If I did it, you can too.

In this Odyssey of Transformation, I have many to thank:

Sylvester Stallone for writing and making the movie "_Rocky_" which changed my life as the fattest kid in my elementary school, Joe Weider of "_Muscle & Fitness_" magazine which I subscribed to during my freshman year in college when I first lived away from home and had to make health choices on my own, Subway Restaurants for their fresh selections when I'm out and about and on the go, all the people at Powerhouse Gym in Ypsilanti, Michigan for providing a healthy culture that encouraged me to make positive changes… and all those people I've encountered who have offered their perspective on dieting, losing fat, and staying happy all throughout life.

And to Dr. David Bressler who told me, "_You can either be right, or you can be happy… not both._" And, "_The only truly happy people I know are those who are creative on a daily basis._" Thank you David. You were right.

Introduction

First and foremost, I should mention that I'm writing this book because the dessert-first dieting mentality worked for me, and I'd like to share it with you... not only so you can transform as I did... but to enjoy your food too.

You see, two years ago, I weighed about 250 pounds with a waist size of 42 inches and a body-fat percentage of 32.4%. As I'm writing this now, my weight is 220 pounds, my pants are slightly below a size 36 waist, and I love the person I see in the mirror... now way below 20% body-fat. In terms of those percentages, I've had them measured via two different methods, including the caliper test, since I joined Powerhouse Gym in October of 2009 just prior to my first book getting published.

Now, I'd like to give you a bit of personal history which I hope provides some confidence in why my counter-intuitive dieting philosophy works.

Please let me add this disclaimer now: I'm not a registered dietician, and I don't have any degrees in nutrition. Nor am I a certified personal trainer or a licensed medical doctor... so use these theories at your own risk with full disclosure that I discovered them via good ol' fashioned common sense.

I learned these techniques the hard way... through lots of trial and error. Sometimes you only learn life's lessons by going through tough times.

Yet, success is on the other side of failure if you don't give up. As I believe Michael Jordan is quoted as saying: "*I miss 100% of the shots I don't take.*"

Many years ago, a movie came out titled, *"Big Mama's House."* While I've never seen it, its title essential describes my household growing up after my parents divorced when I was 8 years old. Food became her escape, and while she doesn't smoke or drink, she *does* love her food. When she smells food cooking... an excitement overtakes her and she's always been one who knows how to make a meal as decadent as possible.

I love her for that.

My mother taught me food is to be savored and enjoyed.

Also, having food in the refrigerator is always a priority for a fat mom... and her kids are sure to reflect that fact in the fat they gain growing up in that kind of environment. I can attest to that fact because I became the fattest kid in my elementary school... by far. She'd say, "*You're just big boned.*"

In junior high, I remember asking out a really cute girl whose locker happened to be next to mine. She politely declined and pointed out the fattest girl in school and suggested I ask her out instead. Needless to say, I was devastated... but not as devastated as when a boy came up, grabbed my big belly, and exclaimed: "*Pinch an inch? Damn, I can pinch a mile!*"

I think I can definitely say that was the low point.

So what changed it?

My grandma took me to go see the movie "*Rocky*" when it was first released. Honestly, seeing that movie changed my life. It made me want to start working out. It made me want to diet. It made me want to win.

Shortly after that, my mom took me to Pro Football Hall of Fame in Canton, Ohio, and I bought a plaque with Vince Lombardi's "*What It Takes to Be Number One*" written on it... which relates how man's finest hour is when he lies on the field of battle exhausted, but victorious.

Looking back, those were the prime components that precipitated my early changes. Yet being that life is full of ebbs and flows like the sinusoid of any waveform, I learned quickly that our body weight and dieting schemes tend to do the same. So my first try at dieting took a *"3 days on, 4 days off"* approach where I tried to be very disciplined three days of the week while giving myself any other four days within the week to splurge.

That turned into Friday food celebrations (6 days of dieting with 1 day off). Then one recent day, a waitress asked, *"Leave any room for dessert?"* That simple question asked at restaurants around the world got me to thinking about the whole fallacy of saying, *"No thanks, I'm on a diet."*

You see, my mom has tried almost single diet under the sun. She's always on some new fangled diet scheme. She never sticks to them. Never has… and probably never will. (sigh…)

Also though, I realized in living with her later in my life that it's just a fact that she'll be coming home with her stash of goodies and junk food. Sometimes she hides it… just like an alcoholic tends to hide their booze. Thus, how do I moderate and balance the steady stream of temptations? Such as at 3am when you're hungry and with the munchies, it's a lot easier to open a bag than to prepare a well-thought-out nutritional meal.

So with that just being a fact of life for me, I had to learn a mindset to not mind all the calorie traps at home. Perhaps that's one reason I prefer to utilize a just-in-time food management approach when it comes down to my own shopping expenditures… because if it's not in the house, I won't eat it.

I learned that you never really stop the reality that we all enjoy food and will continue to do so until the day we die. While you can live without coffee or cigarettes or alcohol or pot or whatever, none of us can live without food.

So why not enjoy it? And then after we do, roll up our sleeves and get back to work eating right.

A bit more personal background for your perspective on me in relation to this new food philosophy concept...

After losing a lot of weight during college and getting a job in Los Angeles as a satellite antenna engineer who played competitive racquetball tournaments, I eventually left that career to become a writer… a screenwriter to be specific because I had an idea for a movie script that causes us to have to face ourselves in the mirror when we need a sign to change towards our destiny. If you'd like to read it, I published it as an eBook titled "*Distortions.*" More than that, its idea caused me to face my own self in the mirror over the years as I've gotten older and learn to love who I saw.

Along the way, I ended up homeless in LA while trying to get an agent to help me sell the finished first draft to Hollywood… which after 9 months of homelessness and sleeping on the beach had me move back home with Mom… where the *Big Mama's House* movie truly took on new meaning.

However, there was one time during those homeless days where I hadn't eaten in days, my energy was almost nil (due to no food to fuel me), and I remember forcing myself to trudge to a homeless foodline in Santa Monica's Palisades Park so I could get a free bite to eat. Needless to say, I was starving and as famished as could be… and I remember when the minister showed up with a bunch of day-old foods that I made myself a baloney sandwich on plain white bread with a huge goop of expired Miracle Whip.

Honestly, I really didn't give a damn about the calorie content of the mayonnaise or that the white bread wasn't whole wheat.

I was just hungry, and it was po' man decadent for being homeless. Let me say: *That was the best fuckin' baloney sandwich I ever ate!*

Please excuse my language there, but I really want to drive down the point of how awesome a plain ol' baloney sandwich tasted that day. It's almost like they say about drugs, "*You're always trying to chase that first high.*"

Then again as *The Zone Diet* mentions in its first pages, *"Food is one of the most powerful drugs you'll ever consume."* I'm loosely paraphrasing the actual wording, but in reading that book while getting into the best shape of my life, I remember that statement hitting home. Its principle is simply to eat a balanced diet... just like grandma always used to say.

In other words, that ol' school sort of thinking often works well. Yet a lot of his theories *do* fit in well with my food philosophy.

So do the philosophies within the book *Eat to Win* because food is fuel. As someone who won many grueling racquetball tournaments, knowing that complex carbs can fuel long endurance performances is worth its weight in gold, and I can attribute such nutritional knowledge for my 1st place wins.

Similarly, the Atkins Diet approach of more lean protein has definitely been a friend of mine in the gym when proteins and amino acids are essential for promoting muscle growth and stimulating consistent calorie consumption as my body rebuilds... kind of what I like to call *"The Caveman Diet."* They needed meat to build strong bones and muscle in order to forage for food. It's a corollary to my *"Camel Diet"* who fuels up in order to cross those extended desert stretches.

While their books are more scientifically based and nutritionally factual, I incorporate a bit of *each* of those three and see this book and my *Dessert First Diet* as more of a way of a lifestyle.

It's the upward spiral way of living... where you take turns using different food philosophy for the specific goals you have immediately at hand. And my approach towards living is assessing and realizing the fact that we all fall off the wagon at one time or another, especially when it comes to tasty food.

Years later, I pondered why that baloney sandwich tasted so damn good. The answer I arrived at was because I was so gosh darned *Hungry*. Simple as that...

Try not eating for days.
Hunger makes you remember.

I guarantee you'll always remember what you chose to eat first
afterwards… and I'll bet too that you truly appreciated it and
enjoyed it more than almost any other time in your life. Being
hungry has that affect.

Yet it also became the premise of what I'm trying to share with
you now… over a decade later… and having just shed over 4
inches from my waist in the process of learning to feed my soul
first… and then diet after.

Discipline needs its downtime.
It's the silences that make the music flow.
It's the spaces between the words that help them make sense.

So if you've stepped on the scale recently and heard yourself
silently say two simple words that start with "*Oh*" and end with
an exclamation point… and if you're tired of the latest diet
trend… allow yourself a bit of disbelief as you embark on this
new food philosophy eBook journey with me. If it worked for
me, it can work for you… you just *have* to *want* to do it. Don't
settle for less than you deserve… because you're worth it.

It's not about being best… but more about doing Our Best.
We're not here for a long time… but for a Good Time.
So let's learn to make every day an excellent one.
Part of it starts by being happy on a daily basis.
Food is a huge ingredient in that equation.

I wish you success in your health…

This is not a diet.
It's a new food philosophy.
The *Dessert First Diet* approach.

Premise

Cure the craving before it blossoms into a binge.
Nip it in the bud.

That is the essence of the *Dessert First Diet* in a nutshell.

Eat the food you want most when it tastes the best.

It advises that devouring a single fresh-baked gooey cookie whose chocolate is still steaming and melty is infinitely better than grazing on a whole box of store-bought cookies that are processed and stale. It's a smarter, rather than harder, approach. The *Dessert First Diet* presents a counter-intuitive technique to foods and feeding your spirit and soul for Life. It advises you to cure any craving before it becomes a binge.

In other words, eat what you want when you're hungriest and when food tastes its best so you nip your craving in the bud, and then go back to work with your nutritional diet. It feels that food is a crucial fuel… not only for body and mind… but for feeding your soul.

It also encourages you to decide on home-cooked meals or food made with love before your hunger forces you to cave in on a bag of store-bought goodies. It's a decision between food that is Alive and that which is dead to some degree on a spiritual level.

This dieting tactic teaches you to savor delicious decadence and enjoy elegant luxury so you can roll up your sleeves and settle into spartan eating smarts when it matters most.

Also though, this new nutritional role-reversal philosophy helped me lose 30 pounds in one year and go from 32.4% bodyfat to a body-mass-index of under 15% while enjoying what I eat when I'm the hungriest… because that's simply when it tastes best. It's also helped me keep it off.

So start to think of "*dessert*" as a verb… not a noun.

It's an active ingredient in satisfying your soul.

The psychology of overeating often comes from an emotional need inside to fill an emptiness that exists in areas other than our actual physical hunger. Sometimes, it just amounts to having a safe place to escape or take the edge off during a difficult day. We all have those days. To deny it is wrong.

Thus, my motto: *Think smarter, not harder.*

That could be retranslated into: *Diet smarter, not harder.*

In other words, any smart man (or woman) can get themselves out of a jam, but it's the intelligent man (or woman) who avoids catastrophe altogether and never needs to extract themselves from delicate or dangerous dilemmas.

So don't think of this as a diet… but instead, a new way of thinking… with a reverse psychology spin on eating tasty treats. If you've seen Woody Allen's movie "*Sleeper*," I think you'll understand the direction I'm coming from. That's a film where he wakes up in the future only to realize that everything he was told was bad is actually good… and vice versa. So if I recall correctly, he learns that eating hot fudge sundaes are healthy.

In moderation of course… as life is always about balance.

Too much of any one thing can also have consequences. If you get burned out from something that's supposed to be good for you, it ceases to be good for you, right?

It's like my mom recently got on a health kick of eating dark chocolate recently because of reports in the news talking up its anti-oxidant prowess… so in cleaning her room a bit, I discovered bags of discarded dark chocolate wrappers. Her mentality being, "*I'll eat myself thin and be healthy too!*"

Good in theory… but simple physics teaches us to consume fewer calories than we burn to lose weight over the long run.

With the myriad of food choices, that's easier said than done.

While I love my mom tremendously, moderation has never been one of her strongest suits or good graces. Yet, she does try… and sometimes that's all that really matters because:

If at first you don't succeed, try, try again!!!

Never give up the battle.
Our dieting is not a sprint.
It's a grueling lifelong marathon.

Pace yourself appropriately.

Consistency

Fate is a function of choice in my opinion.

Everyone has choices. Everyone makes choices.

Even if you choose not to decide, you've still made a choice.

So make good, healthy choices… not bad ones… consistently.

Get your head in this Game of Life.
We *are* goal-oriented people.

But being that it's when I make mistakes that I learn the most, I want you to realize that dieting is a lifetime endeavor. We're in it for the long run… which is why I want you to think of the *Dessert First* approach as a new food philosophy… not a diet.

Yet life's sprints do occur and are necessary… for example, a wedding. But after you're wed, don't abandon ship… otherwise, your spouse may abandon you because you've now turned into someone you weren't when you both legally signed up. In other words, don't be guilty of false advertising.

Balance and moderation in *any* endeavor are crucial for continued success. This is never more important than when it comes down to your own body and your own soul. They are your temple… so to speak.

Consider the following…

Learn the art of multi-tasking so your metabolism burns calories throughout the day. Think of your metabolism like a windmill.

This paradigm shift of the windmill principle is how Lady Gaga's trainer helps keep her in great shape. She eats and exercises in small amounts… all day long. For example, if you can't exercise at a gym for sixty minutes each day, consider sixty 1-minute workouts throughout your entire workday… so you steal moments to take care of yourself.

The windmill principle...

Try to keep it gently spinning all day long… instead of just spinning it fast a few times a day while being stagnant everywhere else. Constant small breezes keep it turning (and burning calories). Now think of those gentle winds as being equivalent to the amounts of food you consume and how often you consume them… so eat more than 3 meals a day for perpetual motion within body and soul. It's like old-fashioned steam locomotives that needed you to constant stoke the engine to get the train down the tracks.

It's only the Conductor at the helm who can keep that train from coming down the tracks… so consider yourself that Conductor… in your very own Symphony of Life.

This idea is nothing new to nutritional analysts with a scientific approach background because they've discovered through detailed measurements that the more you exercise and the more times you eat small meals all throughout the day, the more your metabolism burns in a consistent way.

It's all about maximizing your body's efficiency.

One way to visualize the windmill principle and why eating smaller meals makes sense is to recall anytime you've tried to start a bonfire or when you've sat in front of the fireplace. The larger logs are harder to burn, aren't they? Once they do, they can burn all night (which is an offshoot of my *"Camel Diet"* addendum), but it's the kindling and smaller pieces of wood that help you achieve a roaring fire. The same applies in your stomach. Big meals take a lot longer to digest and for your body to process… while the smaller meals offer less surface area for your stomach's acids to attack.

The *"habit"* of dieting is one of the hardest to acquire in terms of lifelong consistency… life is a sinusoid… ups and downs. But if you make more right choices than wrong ones over the long haul, you while like the results.

So the goal becomes learning to recognize the downswings and to diminish them so you learn to surf your waves of productive eating and metabolizing of calories in a graceful way that makes others want to *hang ten* with you.

However, the momentum you gain when you see results in the mirror and on the scale after diligent discipline and determination? Those are priceless.

Why? Because you **_earn_** them.

You don't buy them.

You earn 'em.

That ol' fashioned thing called *"hard work"* that so many people tend to forget when they think they can buy a pill instead or hire a plastic surgeon for some cosmetic nips and tucks to reach their physical appearance goals. The problem with that approach is that to the eagle eye, it always looks fake. The *"pill for everything"* approach doesn't always work.

That's why this dieting approach is about acknowledging that cravings are a fact of life… and to get back on the wagon after you've enjoyed a pit stop to refuel your gumption to get your mojo workin' once again – *consistently*.

Dessert-First…
It's not really a *Diet*.
It's a <u>new food philosophy</u>.

Food as Fuel

When I joined Powerhouse Gym in October of 2009, I bought a 6-month package that included a digital physical assessment of my health. At the time, I was 41 years old with 32.4% body-fat, and the machine's analysis told me I had the Real Age of a 49 year old. Six months later when I renewed my member and had another analysis, I was amazed at the fact that I'd actually gained weight (10 pounds), but that I'd dropped 10% in my BMI (body-mass-index) along the way. So the weight I'd gained was muscle while the fat had melted away. I suggested it was my eating habits changing as well as my training rituals as well.

It was at that point that the trainer who I selected to do the assessment mentioned something that stuck: "Yeah, *food is a crucial fuel.*"

Being that he had just slimmed down for a bodybuilding competition, I firmly found his quick quip to be 100% accurate. That's the reason I selected him to do the analysis. I'd watched him diet down while training more intensely than I'd ever seen anyone work out in a while.

That's also extremely similar to Barry Sears assertion that *food is the most powerful drug you will ever consume.* If you want just the gist of Dr. Sears' book *"The Zone Diet,"* that'd be it. He offered another important lesson I learned to incorporate:

Shop around the edges of a grocery store.
The center of the store is where the fat is at.

Try it sometime and see just exactly what you can buy on the perimeter of a grocery store… because it's once you start walking down the actual aisles that your eventual diet will go into the danger zone of too much calorie consumption – *of the wrong calories you want to consume!*

It's not that they're bad foods. It's just that they have a higher tendency to make you heavy… those down the aisles rather than around the perimeter of any grocery store. The aisles tend to have all the highly refined stuff in boxes and bags that tend to be processed to some degree.

Those don't provide the same *fuel* as those fresh foods on the outside edge.

One of my favorite Arnold Schwarzenegger quotes from his *"Pumping Iron"* film is when he talks about being a sculptor. Back then, he was sculpting his body to become the world champion bodybuilder who became the Hollywood mega-star and eventual governor of California.

Another thing from that film and era that stuck with me is that *"you don't put junk fuel in a Maserati."*

If your body is that sports car, what kind of gas do you fill it with? The cheap stuff or premium? Also, do you keep such a precision automobile highly tuned for peak performance when it matters most? Next question: If you were a car, what kind of car would you be? A Lamborghini or an Edsel?

Food for thought…

A Binge Society

The movie *"Wall Street"* and Gordon Gekko's *"Greed is good"* mentality have definitely had a trickle-down effect on society. By making them aware of such concepts, a part of all of us runs with it to some extent. It's like *if some is good, more is better* has become somewhat of a mantra for us.

Thus, if something is considered healthy, a part of us overindulges in it to maximize the benefit. Is that correct thinking? I think not.

It's the ol' lesson of finding out about a new diet super food… and then thinking that eating a few cases of 'em will slim us down real good.

Sigh…

Remember. It doesn't matter how good a food is for you, if you consume too many calories on any given day, no matter how healthy they may be perceived, you *will* gain weight – period. Simple physics says so.

So does our scale at the doctor's office.

That's one frustrating thing I've encountered in living at *Big Mama's House*. She tends to get angry if I hold up a mirror of some sort to her… letting her know that she needs to change her consumption and purchasing habits… and then goes and pays a doctor at the hospital to hear the same exact thing.

It's a case of "please *don't shoot me, I'm just the messenger."*

How often do we listen to those cosmic messengers when God sends 'em… because He does? Trust and believe that! He likes to send warning shots across our bow to see if we'll make a change.

And if we don't?

Beware.

Don't shoot the messenger… especially in this binge society that thinks more is better. Sometimes, more is just simply more… especially around our waistlines.

I'm not sure why my Mom has this innate desire for a full refrigerator. She likes buying food in bulk… or as I often like to say: *"Going into debt by **saving** money."* If you buy so much food that some of it spoils and needs to be thrown away, then all those saving really don't mean a darn, do they?

For instance, as I'm writing this, it's Thanksgiving week of 2011. So Mom went about bought two turkeys (because they were on sale), a bunch of marked down food (because they're close to their expiration dates), an entire cheesecake, and a new girdle (apparently to strap it all in). In the process of all these perceived savings, I noticed that she proceeded to bounce her bank account… because she shopped without knowing of her bank account's balance. So the savings actually cost us more.

The Lord's *"Serenity"* prayer definitely comes in handy for times like these, and I have to silently remind myself that food wasn't always this plentiful… *"Lord, grant me to serenity to accept the things I can not change, the courage to change the things I can, and the wisdom to know the difference."*

You can either be right, or you can be happy… not both.

Yet a bounced bank account means no savings at the store.

And the girdle and the expired cheesecake aren't helping any.

Don't get me wrong; I love my mother tremendously. It's just sometimes I don't understand the rationale. Perhaps it's the credit card society we're being inundated with more and more these days of instant gratification and planned obsolescence so we have to buy – buy – buy.

Another thing to consider when changing your habits that hanging around people who eat junk food plants a seed that soon blossoms into a binge.

That's one thing any recovering addict has to learn.
They need to learn to make new friends for growth.
If you don't, those enablers pull you down and under.

Once distance is established from such similar addicts (of any sort), you see with a hindsight power of observation that provides a sentient clarity.

One thing I've started doing is going to grocery stores and actively look inside people's baskets and shopping carts. Then I assess who's pushing the cart to see if their food choices align with their body-type.

They always do.

Always.

So don't put all your eggs in one basket y'all.

Also, I noticed that obese people usually had shopping carts stuffed to the gills… while thin people tended to buy what they needed for the night.

That's why I mention the just-in-time principle to many… buy when you need it and desire it most… and even then just buy what you need and not what you want. The two are usually disparagingly different.

Doing that, looking inside people's carts, actually came to me in 1997 and the beginning of 1998 when I worked as a full-service gas station attendant in Seattle on the graveyard shift… right below the Space Needle.

I had just finished the first draft of my "*Distortions*" screenplay which uses mirrors as a supernatural portal that shows us our Inner Truth. After completing that epic ensemble supernatural rock opera, I felt a vacuum. I did what I set out to do after cocooning myself for months and needed to get back out into the world… and I learned: *people do need people*.

In hindsight, I think I can honestly say that it was one of the best jobs of my life because from 11pm through 7am, I'd see the entire spectrum of humanity… simply because almost everyone needs gas… or a 24-hour store in the middle of the downtown district where they tend to be scarce.

You see, I'd see people from all walks of life in timely ritualistic living, and being that my job allowed me unspoken permission to approach people's cars, look inside as they opened their wallets or purses, and spend time pumping their gas and washing their windshields, Life provided me with a crash course in Current Culture Anthropology 101 by being a gas pumper.

I'd keep myself amused during the down times by quoting lines to myself from Steve Martin's "*The Jerk*" like, "*He hates these cans!*" and "*Step right up, take a chance, and win some crap!*" and his other movie quote: "*I need this… and that's all I need.*"

When you start talking to yourself to keep you amused, life gets interesting. When you start answering yourself, people call a doctor. But to me, it's just an integral component of being a writer… hearing your characters speak. As I once heard about one author, he said that his characters came to him and told him, "*You've created us. We demand more story!*"

Getting back though…

You'd be amazed at how much the inside of a car, wallet, or purse reveals about a person. Are they messy? Are they clean? What do they keep in their wallet? Is the money messy or in order? What does their car or truck smell like? Have they washed their vehicle recently? Are they suspicious that I'm asking to assist them? Do they want to do it themselves instead of letting me? Do they tip? If so, are they generous and consistent tippers? Do they notice or appreciate the care I take and the pride I place in my job... no matter how lowly it may seem to them?

The same lessons apply when I go into a grocery store and look inside people's shopping carts, see how they pay (cash, credit, coupons, and/or food stamps), see who they bring along with them, watch what they purchase and if they're embarrassed buying it... as all those factors are indicators that reveal much for sales and marketing types... those who *want* you to use their food or gas cards... so they can track your times, your purchases, your trends. Statistical trends do predict patterns.

The reasoning for learning to look at these things is similar to working at the gas station... just as people need gas for our cars, we all need food too.

So consider being more observant of others... so you can see yourself and your buying patterns with a bit more transparency. It may enable you to make changes that can assist you in living a healthier overall lifestyle.

Sometimes we need to see ourselves in the mirror with fresh eyes. An example of this is that this morning, I read a draft of a screenplay I completed in 2009... which I finished the first draft for in 1997. Also to note is that in 2010, I paid someone to read both drafts and was hurt by their assessment that some crucial edge had been lost in the translation from the first version to the last one in 2009. To me, it was an insult... and I ended the relationship abruptly. It's a case where my true friends tell me the things I really don't want to hear.

The same applies when someone may say you need to lose weight. They really aren't trying to hurt you. They're just trying to help. But brutal honesty often isn't always the best route to travel.

Yet it really does help somewhere along the line because that
one drop of truth shatters an ego and resonates… and maybe
that ego needed a crack or two in it. Because that may be the
opening that allows the spirit to enter… the spirit of change…
and being able to see yourself from a different and fresh
perspective… where you may have been a bit blinded before.

So in getting back to the 2009 version of my screenplay, I read it
this morning (the week of Thanksgiving 2011) after having lost
weight from my peak obesity in October of 2009. And it was
interesting that being leaner helped me realize how overly-
verbose my 2009 dialogue was. It was as if I was spoonfeeding
every thought to the reader… instead of letting body language
and subtle cues speak for themselves. In other words, a picture
can say a thousand words… and I then realized that my script
consultant was right.

Less tends to be more… that's the lesson I learned.

Not only in writing, in soundbytes, in eating… but in Life, in
general. Some ideas to ponder as you view your true self in the
mirror and think about how you'd like to sculpt yourself.

Just remember that hindsight often reveals all with that Oprah
A-Ha Moment which makes us smile up at the sky and now
know why God works in mysterious ways that are often slow…
so the roots grow strong and deep.

As a Catholic, one thought I want to end this chapter on is the
idea of giving up things for Lent. On Fat Tuesday, everyone
likes to party Mardi-Gras-style prior to Ash Wednesday's
resolution to abstain from whatever bad habit you choose to do
without. The thing is… once Easter arrives and after the Lenten
resolutions are permitted to be gone, are you willing to pick up
the *old* habit/addiction again? Remember. One is too many. A
million is never enough. Get a taste for that ol' familiar habit
and you may regret it.

One last thing I should mention about binges: You often acquire the habits of those you date or live with. If you live with someone who lacks self-control, it often gets incorporated into your everyday life too.

That's one reason I think a lot of people get divorced after marrying early. One partner in the marriage desires to make a change while the other does not. In electrical engineering terms, it creates an *impedance mismatch*. In waveguide and antenna theory, it sets up a high *standing-wave ratio* where the feedback loop between opposing parties gets to the point of overloading and frying each other's circuit boards… to the point where irreconcilable differences become an easy reason for a judge to grant the divorce.

Some more food for thought as we desire changes in each other and in our selves… if you change for the better and your spouse doesn't can you still live with each other? Can a smoker and a non-smoker survive together? The same is true with dieting and exercise. We become like those we associate with.

Something to think about…

Cure the Craving

In trying out this *Dessert First Diet* philosophy on myself, the one thing I've kept in mind is that eating a delicious single serving is always better than buying the whole box. If you bring it home, chances are you'll eat it.

It's as simple as that.

That's also the reason I don't keep a stocked bar at my home. If I buy huge amounts of beer, wine, and liquor, I know myself well enough to know that I tend to overindulge and drink it a lot faster than I should. And trust me; I've had the hangover headaches to prove it. It's a part of being in Big Mama's House… you tend to take on an addictive personality. Not part of the plan… just part of the truth… and it takes facing the truth to make a positive change.

Part of the cure is to realize this… and to shop accordingly.

Just know… it's a lot harder to go to the store when a craving strikes than it is to walk into the kitchen an open the cupboard. If it's not handy, you're a whole lot less likely to gather the gumption to go out and consume it.

In other words, our society teaches us to forage for food all at once… rather than the healthier just-in-time mentality of eating as you go.

Remember that cravings *will* gnaw at the back of your mind until you take the time to cure them. In my opinion, better sooner than later. Nip them in the bud. Then get back to work on more important stuff with bigger fish to fry. Another way of looking at it is to not sweat the small stuff and to recall that it all tends to be small stuff when you really get down to it.

So if you're constantly and consistently super-sizing your meal, you will eventually super-size yourself… plain and simple.

Even think about using smaller dishes and plates… seriously.

If your mind sees a small serving, it becomes less hungry.
It's an offshoot of the placebo effect - mind over matter.

And when you get down to it, matter don't matter.

Another way of dieting down is to ditch the distractions while
eating. Keep your focus on your food… and SLOW DOWN.
You don't need to eat it all in one big gulp. By taking your time
and letting food digest, you tend to find yourself fuller on less
calories. That's because you absorb the food and actually
realize that you didn't need as much as you thought you did.

Sometimes it takes two steps back to make three leaps forward.

An idea that supermodel Yasmeen Ghauri advised in a 1997
magazine article was to try to eat while sitting down rather than
standing up. Since taking her advice, I've come to realize how
much her sage wisdom is right. Sitting down with a meal and
no TV makes it so much more satisfying.

Analyze your schedule to dictate how big of a meal to eat.
When will you have time to sit down and eat again? You must
sit in order to savor… so you're not just cramming in food on
the go (a big no-no).

Realize that a meal consisting of many small plates doesn't
always satisfy. That's one thing to consider too… eating like a
camel… because you don't always know when you're going to
be able to eat again.

Again, more food for thought…

Food that is Alive

Recently while writing this book, my mom's 93 year old friend, Nellie, had to go to the hospital because of extremely high blood pressure. In the course of her doctor's treatment, part of his advice was to eat more yogurt than usual because of the active cultures would help her stomach (part of which she had removed due to a past cancer). His rationale is that yogurt is Alive.

The fact is though that Nellie called, and as I answered, all she could do was complain how she'd gotten fed up with yogurt after days of eating it consistently saying: "*After I get better, I don't wanna see another cup of yogurt all my life! If I eat one more cup, I think I'm gonna throw up.*"

That's one nice thing I love about good ol' Nellie; she calls 'em as she sees 'em. At her age, why beat around the bush with a bunch of BS? She doesn't mince words, and why would she need to? At 93, she's earned her latitude.

One thing I love about her is when she cooks. Because when she does, she makes so much food cooked with her special brand of love that she gives a lot of it to me... and her cookin', made with loving care, tastes damn good.

To me, it's all about the fact that she cares about every ingredient she adds.

Years ago in 1997 when I lived in Seattle, I invited a homeless man to come over and stay a day or two... allowing him to wash his clothes and get some sleep with the peace of mind of not having to keep that inner eye awake in case of the emergencies that sleeping on the streets present. As I barbequed some steak and chicken for us, I remember how much he appreciated the fact that I was cooking for him... and not just buying some stuff from the store. As we watched the Puget Sound sunset on my balcony while eating strawberry ice cream (his favorite), he told me why the food tasted so good:

"The food you made... tastes good... because it's Alive."

One of the reasons I helped him is because I knew he'd had a stroke months earlier and needed a friend. Likewise, because being that I moved to Seattle to scout locations for my film, *"Distortions,"* I didn't know anyone. Also though, I wanted to go to a place where people weren't telling me *"You can't"* and instead told me *"You can"* simply because they didn't know me.

Helping him get back Home, to me, was like living through the movie *"Rain Man,"* and I later found funny others would do the same for me in 1999.

Little did I know that I'd be homeless two years later trying to sell that movie to Hollywood, but Bobby's comment about *"being Alive"* definitely resonated... as did his remark about why he liked the jean jacket I gave him:

"Pockets!"

For a homeless man, pockets can be priceless.

Unfortunately, I had to learn that lesson too... the hard way.

Yet years later, I'm glad to say that those schools of hard knocks helped me to learn things school doesn't teach. If anything, it makes you appreciate the good things when they arrive... and to be grateful for them.

Thus, on Thanksgiving Day 2011 as I write this, I was pleased with a quick quip one of the guys at Powerhouse Gym told me on his way out for the day: *"Just makin' the down-payment on the calorie debt I'm about to incur later today at Thanksgiving Dinner with The (Parental) Units."*

It's precious improv lines like that which make life worth living... but then, so are Thanksgiving meals that mean more because they're made with love.

During the holiday season though of Thanksgiving to the New Year, just know that this is the most tempting time of the year when it comes to food, and sometimes it pays to put this *Dessert First Diet* advice to work by allowing yourself to indulge in the things you've waited all year for… such as pumpkin pie by biting the bullet, saying WTF, and getting back to work.

Balance and moderation work better with mini-rewards.

Those carrots at the end of the stick sometimes do the trick.

Tricks of the trade: Try a maple syrup drizzle over a Caesar salad… so a spoonful of sugar helps the medicine go down. It makes you look forward to a good salad. I'm amazed at how much further a tiny bit of maple syrup will go on a salad as compared to some oatmeal (which absorbs the tasty topping instead of having it spread around like on lettuce leafs).

Also, the maple syrup is a more natural sugar than sucrose or dextrose. And to me, whatever mankind cleaves has side-effects. That's why an au natural approach which appreciates living foods made with loving care works.

For example, if you're forced to decide between butter and margarine, choose the butter… because it's more natural than that fake crap they try to pass off as being better for you. To me, that's just their marketing machine working in overdrive trying to sell you things you really don't need. Watch late night TV advertising with all the infomercials and you'll get my point.

The thing to analyze and assess with any new diet fad is this: "*Is it sustainable? Will it work over the long haul?*" If not, ditch it.

Just trying to throw out an idea or two you may want to run with in your own everyday attempts to build a better body. More natural food tends to have a "*living*" sense to it that feeds the soul. As my homeless friend said, "*I like it because it's Alive.*"

White Bread Buns

Dr. Joel Fuhrman, M.D. suggests that health equates to the ratio of nutrients to calories in the foods you consume. He says that fat melts away when the foods you consume are nutrient-dense.

Dr. Oz on TV suggests that processed foods (like pasta, white rice, and white bread) and fried foods are *"the new cocaine"* in the obesity epidemic. They satisfy fast but leave you empty quickly. In other words, they offer a *"high"* and produce a quick crash that leaves you craving more and more with an intense need to fuel the craving with a blossoming binge. Highly refined carbs are metaphorically similar to cocaine. They give you a rush of serotonin and dopamine that messes up your hormones and endorphins with the fast rush they produce.

Also, I always find it interesting how some of the principles I learned in physics and electrical engineering apply in other areas. For example, I remember teaching a lab course in grad school at the University of Michigan about digital operational amplifiers where we taught the students that the gain-bandwidth product is always a constant.

Thus, if you have a high gain, your frequency bandwidth will be narrow… and vice versa, a large spectrum of bandwidth will only give you a low gain to amplify your device.

The same applies with drugs which is why cocaine is such a high *"high"* and a quick crash leaving you craving more… immediately… and food too (such as the highly refined processed foods that Dr. Oz calls *"The New Cocaine"*).

So always keep in the mind the amount of nutrients and the reason you're eating the foods you are. Is it because you need a quick burst of energy to get over that tired hump and slump? Or is it because you have a long journey ahead and aren't sure when your next camel-like meal will be.

Sometimes we do have a desert to cross.
Gain-bandwidth equals a constant.
Apply it to the foods you choose.

Fundamental laws of the universe apply in all areas… that's one
reason I think Jesus spoke so often in parables and metaphors:
*"If you can help them visualize it, you can teach them the
underlying principles."* Give them a taste with the appetizer so
they will want the main course.

Processed, refined foods have all the nutrients knocked out of
them. Similarly, overcooking vegetables eliminates the vitamin
content. My mom is notorious for this. She loves to heat
everything on high so it gets done faster. Thus, al dente is not in
her cooking vocabulary. She tends to bleach out all the
nutrients, vitamins, and minerals in the process. If you're
cooking the color out of the food, you're draining all the
benefits that go along with your particular meal selection.

It's a penny-wise, pound-foolish way of cooking.
Shop smarter so you don't have to work out harder.

Like a nickel holding up a dime, don't double-deed your
exercise needs. That way after you've only got a quarter of the
way to go to reach your goal, you don't have to stop and ask
when you're a dime's worth away.

Another active eating technique I want you to try is when you
go out for a burger and a beer; take off the bun that doesn't have
any sauce or cheese on it. Don't eat it. They're unnecessary
calories. If it doesn't have any of the interesting stuff on it, it's
really there to keep your hands dry. So maybe use the lettuce as
the opposing bun instead. Just less calories to burn off later.

Next, try to eat the burger and fixin's first, and then round out
your meal with the French fries after. While people may argue
that the burger's saturated fat is bad, it still packs a lot of good
ol' fashioned protein that would make a caveman proud. Really,
it's the fried potatoes we call fries that are the emptiest of all the

calories on that particular plate. At least with the beer, you get a bit of a buzz bang for your buck. So burger first, fries last. A restaurant burger's bun is typically just a hockey puck of empty calories. Filler. Also, it's ratio of nutrients to calories just doesn't make the cut.

A similar theory is the price breaks people offer you as an enticement to get your business. For example, my chiropractor was telling me of a stretch when he'd wait to eat so he could travel 20 miles to take advantage of a $2 ice cream shake that felt as if it weighed 2 pounds that you literally had to eat with a spoon and was a meal in and of itself. The problem is, he'd eat it at 2pm and then have a 5pm crash because of the lack of nutrients in proportion to the amount of calories he consumed while trying to save money as he enjoyed a shake that ate like a meal. The other conundrum he didn't realize is that at $4/gallon for gasoline, the 40 mile roundtrip actually made that shake cost $10, not $2… on top of the fact that it caused him to crash and added calories without nutrients.

That's the thing, lower prices are being offered more and more if you buy more… and more often. This frequently leads to weight gain because it entices you to indulge in larger portions in one single sitting that are harder for your stomach to burn off over the course of the day.

One last thing I'd like to add for you to consider in this chapter: Smaller plate sizes promote smaller amounts consumed at a single sitting.

If your smaller plate is filled, while your larger plate looks empty (even though they contain the exact same amount of food), your mind plays a trick on you in thinking and telling you that you're not getting the same amount of satisfaction from what you eat. Thus, use smaller plates and bowls.

It's a placebo effect sort of approach to plate-size choices.

Feeding Your Soul

When it comes to feeding your soul, always consider whether your choice feeds a need you've had in the back of your mind for a while.

Then try to clear it *"off the stack."*

Clear the clutter in your mind.

The closer to natural form the food is, the healthier it tends to be. Therefore, the first ingredient in the foods and grains you buy should be precipitated by the word: WHOLE. For example: whole wheat bread.

Recently, I heard a person compare Trader Joes to Whole Foods, and he quipped about the latter: *"Oh, you mean Whole Paycheck?"* I had to laugh. Organic foods do tend to be more expensive. And while they're not 100% necessary, if you can afford them, I'd recommend them. Being more pesticide-free and naturally-handled is always a smarter choice.

Another thing to consider is that protein-rich breakfast tends to keep you fuller longer while being a better fuel for productivity. Again, it's a case of the ratio of nutrients to calories helping you fuel your morning. Assess what is stoking your engine as your steam train tries to chug down the tracks. Being the conductor at the helm, how do you get it going?

Is it an empty caffeinated beverage or is it a nutrient rich meal? The fact is, we get so ingrained to *thinking* we *need* caffeine that we don't know how to go without it. I recently conducted an experiment on myself where I purposely went caffeine-free for two weeks, and I found that I really didn't need it as much of it as I thought to get going. Then when I had a coffee, I almost felt unsafe to drive because I was so *wired*. Since succumbing to such a legal and accepted habit, I'm addicted once again.

In this wirelessly wired world, maybe that's what they want.
One can be too many, and a million never tends to be enough.

Sigh…

Also, I recently read how those who eat breakfast tend to stay
slimmer over time simply because they start stoking their
metabolism's engine early… rather than having it go into
ketosis and storing fat because of going it starvation mode of
trying to save itself. For example, I recently heard of a 500
calorie per day diet, and the TV reporter interviewed a
nutritionist who said that our brains *alone* require 600 calories a
day to survive… so those who are only eating 500 calories each
day are actually losing weight from loss of weight in muscle and
vital organs… certainly not a soulful approach.

Consider dining in more often… simply since you can control
the ingredients a lot easier than you can at a restaurant or out
and about.

Incorporate fruits, vegetables, and produce at *every* meal.
The more colorful your meals, the healthier they tend to be.

Just remember, if God gave it to us naturally, it has a higher
tendency to fill us on a soulful level. That's why coca leaves
aren't the addiction that cocaine is. It's all about how mankind
cleaves it and distills or processes it that leads to those nasty
side-effects that tend to lead the soul down destructive paths.

Having lived through such destructive detours in my life and
recovered enough to know to *just say no*, I can honestly say
ignorance can often be bliss when someone offers something
new to you for free. You don't always have to take the freebie.

Always ask before indulging: What are the long-term side-
effects? Is this something my soul can handle if I happen to like
it a lot? If not, just say *"no thanks"* and politely walk the other
way. Just because it's offered for free doesn't mean you need it.

Retraining the Palette

When I was speaking with a woman recently who was taking a
class on everyday nutrition, she brought up the concept of how
consciously being aware of calorie proportions makes it easier
to retrain yourself in eating right when it matters most. She had
just had a baby and was trying to lose the baby fat she'd gained.
Over the next few months, it was amazing to see her diet down
with such a conscious food philosophy.

Her dad mentioned, _"I'd rather trust the martial artist who
practiced one kick a thousand times rather than the person who
tries a thousand kicks once."_ My mom refers to it as: _jack of all
trades – master of none._

In other words, develop muscle memory.

Another way to look at it is to develop _"taste memory"_… where
you can taste something and know if the ingredients disagree
with you. She also mentioned how once you've changed your
eating habits, you begin to notice the taste of hidden additives
much quicker. She's right.

If you cut sugar out of your diet, it becomes easy to taste sweet
treats fast. Also, if they are sweet, you can sense if it's an
artificially sweetness too.

It's similar to being in a room with a smoker after you've quit
smoking. Once you leave, you notice the smell of the smoke on
your clothes. Before you quit, you don't notice because your
senses are dulled to the culprit.

So try to retrain yourself to _"taste"_ again before swallowing.

How many times do you chew your food before gulping it
down? I learned this from watching my dad eat. He was one of
eight kids… so if he didn't eat fast and was still hungry, he
didn't get second helpings. He learned _"fast eating"_ as a kid

simply because food was scarce back then for him. It's a habit that's stayed with him into his later years.

It's also one that I've consciously had to *un*learn.

The same applies with retraining your palette and the way you eat. Sometimes we don't really realize how we eat or what we're really eating. We just do it because that's the way we were raised. Those kind of environmental habitual rituals are often the hardest to break and retrain.

Start trying to taste the actual individual ingredients... similar to an undercover cop tasting or smelling drugs to see if they're the real deal.

A similar concept is what I call *The Zen of Yard Cleaning –* "*Weeding my garden... to help it grow.*" To me, not enough people weed their metaphorical gardens. By not doing so, the weeds choke out the good stuff of the nutrients they need to grow up strong and healthy.

There's a gospel parable that discusses the same fact, but it also applies directly to our diets and the foods we choose to fuel us up. Consider junk food and fast food to be those weeds that need weeding out of your everyday diet. Are they choking your health from truly thriving? Think about how many times you eat out. Can you do better?

I remember being in a courtroom once years ago and hearing a case where this woman was merging onto a highway and cut someone off by speeding up... and got a ticket. When she explained her side of the story, the judge admonished her by saying, "*You can always go slower.*" He's right... not just about driving... but about Life in general. We can always slow down.

If we're always at a digital state of one, what do you do to get back to zero?

What do we do to recharge our internal battery? Because once you burn out from information overload, regaining gumption is totally tougher than ever before. The same is true with exercising overload... which is usually when Life slows you down with an injury that makes you *wish* you slowed down sooner rather than being forced to later on.

Retraining yourself to think smarter and not harder takes time... but it *is* worth it. It's a paradigm shift we all need to make.

"Leave the gun; take the cannoli." How many of you have quoted that line from *The Godfather*? The thing is... when you've ate a cannoli, have you ever taken the time to realize how heavy and hefty one of those babies are? I'm not speaking about the calorie content either... but just feeling the literal weight that presents itself when you hold one in your hand.

Heavy cream is *heavy*.

It *does* taste good though.

And *that* is the conundrum.

Consider doing that for everything you eat. Subconsciously weigh it in your hand before you decide to eat it... or before you decide how much of it to eat. If it weighs X amount, you'll have to burn that amount of weight off before getting back to where you started before devouring it.

It's one way of retraining your palette... consciously realizing how much something weighs and its ratio of calories to nutrients before you take a bite.

Sometimes, I've even started chewing on a tasteless mouthful of food because of mindless grazing... and then realized how many calories I was about to consume... and spit it out before I swallowed it. It's not exactly bulimic binging and purging, but it *is* becoming *aware* of what I *want* versus what I truly *need* before ingesting it fully and then having to process it off.

For example, many months ago I decided to order a pizza for delivery… one of those really decadent ones with tons of toppings. Needless to say, it weighed a ton when it arrived, but being late at night and really, really hungry, I didn't care and devoured it all. Boy, did I pay the price for it the very next day… as well as in days to come in realizing how much that one simple pizza put me behind in my weight loss and fitness goals.

It becomes an issue of what I call "*active eating*" – such as pulling off fried flakes that contain no meat when you've got a hankering for fried food. Only eat the good stuff with protein inside and try to avoid as much of the fried excess as possible… in other words, beware of hidden calorie traps.

Become a consciously active eater.
Retrain yourself and your taste palette.
Your figure and waistline will thank you for it.

Trust me…

All things in moderation.

Fast Food Conundrum

So what are we to do when we're out and about and trying to grab a quick bite? Beef jerky is always good… but heavy in sodium. Nuts can be a good choice but they're typically over-salted too with many of their calories coming from fat… good fat, mind you… but a gram of fat consists of 9 calories versus 4 calories in each gram of protein and/or carbohydrate.

In the past, fast food has been a nutritional wasteland.

Lately though, Subway has been the exception.

They provide a selection of healthy choices.

The only problem is… you have to be willing to make those smart selections when there are so many choices to choose from at any Subway. For example, they have a ton of fresh-baked buns. Do you get wheat? Also, after you have your meat and vegetables, do you add a sauce, salt, and pepper? The sodium in the salt really isn't necessary, and I'm always surprised that the prep people are surprised when I don't get any sauce on my sandwich. I guess I'm the exception… because in my opinion, all the sauces just add unnecessary calories I have to go and burn off later on.

I once heard a professional poker player saying that his first job was with Subway… calling himself: *"A sandwich artiste."* The announcer quipped, *"Ah, the Picasso of Cold Cuts."*

Myself, my first real job was for McDonalds. Interestingly enough, I recently learned that the obese owner of that particular store passed away a few years ago… so you might consider that he might have died eating his own food. It's a possibility.

That's the topic of the film documentary titled, *"Supersize Me."* If you've never seen it, I highly recommend it. It follows the narrator as he eats a supersize meal 3-4 times a day for a month.

The results are shocking. To see the before and after photos, cholesterol levels, and blood pressure readings from following such a diet to the extreme *will* make you rethink your decision to make that trip through any fast food drive-thru window.

But then that's the whole point of why he made the film.

Sometimes more isn't better. Sometimes more is just more.

Start to be active in making the *less is more* paradigm shift.

And actually, films like that have caused fast-food chains like McDonalds to start offering healthier alternatives on their menus. The fact is though, we have to be willing to buy them when we're on the run and getting a meal at the drive-thru. McDonalds isn't the culprit, *we are* for making bad choices.

It's like, try going into a donut shop for a simple sandwich. Such visual temptation and fried pastry aromas invite you to add-on a donut too.

So if you do decide to devour that fresh donut, consider only eating the frosting off the top. Then throw away the rest of the donut that is less "*interesting*" to eat... less time on the treadmill to burn off your detour into delicious decadence. Or better yet, give the rest to the birds. They tend to be hungry and looking for food... and, to me, it builds up *birdy karma*.

Do onto others as you want done onto you... the golden rule... especially when it comes down to all God's creatures.

Feeding hungry bellies always makes for a wiser and more appreciatively compassionate soul.

That's where those hockey pucks of white bread buns make others happy... because you *can* give them away to animals who can't feed themselves like we can because of evolution's invention of opposable thumbs.

My mom has told me repeatedly that I'd always want to tear off my crusts from the bread and give them to the birds. She says she doesn't know where I got that from but insists that it just came naturally. It makes me glad.

Anyways, so consider skimming those tasty tops… just like skim milk gets its artery-clogging creamy saturated fats removed with one quick scoop.

Fast food is fun.

But make it a treat… or a reward… not an everyday thing.

As the Dalai Lama recently said about what confounds him about mankind, his response was, "*Man. Because he sacrifices his health in order to make money… and then sacrifices money to recuperate his health.*"

Amen, my friend… amen.

The Wide Variety of Sugars

Sugar comes in many forms and many corporations who profit from these types of food try to hide the fact that you're consuming a lot of sugar or hidden sodium (like juice drinks and microwave dinners for example). To me, it's yet another instance of *"bait and switch"* tactics from the food industry. Don't be hoodwinked. Frankenfoods can kill you just as well as those cancer sticks people call cigarettes.

Eat your fruits; don't drink them in a juice or a fruit cocktail.

Read the back of any regular soda label or ingredients for a processed dessert… and you'll find all kinds of crazy names for sugar. I often wonder who gets to make up those artificial names anyways.

Now, they even sell *"throw back"* sodas that use real sugar… for that *"back in the day"* kind of taste of ol' school sugar water. Sucrose, dextrose, white sugar, brown sugar, artificial sweeteners with ingredient names you can't even pronounce… is that what you really need?

For example, as I read my diet soda label, it says: *"Phenylketonurics: contains phenylalanine."* WTF are those?!? I don't know, but I tend to drink 'em almost every day. Notice that the last word has a *lala* syllable in it… putting you in la-la land, I presume. You are what you eat, right? So that's why I must eat so many nuts. (haha!)

Taking note of such artificial ingredients is often the first step.

Think about them enough, and you'll soon say: *"I don't need 'em."* Something that looks good may not be the best for you… remember that. As my racquetball coach used to say: *"Good from far, but far from good."*

Yet the thing to keep in mind when you've got a sweet tooth is that the more natural the sugars, the better off you are. Maple syrup is a good example. It's a lot better choice for a sense of sweetness than other alternatives.

One of my friends explains that artificial sweeteners are meant to bombard your taste buds with too much fake sweetness… arguing that it fools your mind and body into thinking its full… when it's really not… so I get scolded anytime I drink a diet soda. It's like it teases your body into thinking its getting a lot of sugar calories… dulling down your sense of taste. Again, you need to retrain your palette to do without it. One healthy alternative is sparkling water… only, that's not nearly as accessible at your corner store as soda pop… so buy it in bulk if you do decide to make the switch.

Another instance is when I hear commercials for ginger ale tout: *"Made with real ginger!"* It's yet another case of *"eat your ginger, don't drink it."*

Those snake-oil salesmen have gotten savvier over the years.

That doesn't mean you have to buy from them though.

Just be aware that they exist and say *"No thanks."*

Eating When Food Tastes Best

One of the bonuses of this *Dessert First Diet* philosophy is that you allow yourself to eat what you're craving when you're hungriest... which is also when food tastes its best. That's the reverse psychology at work again... because if you save dessert for last, chances are you won't enjoy it as much since you're already full. The key to my approach is to feed your soul.

Then make healthier food choices after the indulgence... which provides a more well-rounded diet that also satisfies our innate desires for tasty treats.

Then get back to work after the mini-binge. Simple as that.

Recently, I watched a local news report where the zoo was giving polar bears *"special"* pizza... with tons of sardines, anchovies, and other toppings only a bear would find delicious. The weatherman's quip was, *"Ah, put enough cheese on it, and you'd never know the difference."*

Like they say, *"One person's trash is another person's treasure."* Or, *"Beauty is in the eye of the beholder."*

If you are going to follow this new-fangled, cockamamie *Dessert First Diet* approach of mine, one idea I recommend to keep in mind is to try and eat the most early on and then taper down the size of your meals as the day progresses so your body has time to burn what's been eaten before you fall asleep.

As many will remind you: those late night snacks hurt the most.

That's simply since your sleeping body burns calories slower.

Hibernation mode has you retain calories... but on the other hand, a full belly can provide an awesome night of sleep better than a growling stomach can any day and any night. So try to balance both for the immediate need at hand... and don't scold yourself too much if you need that decadent delight when the late night munchies strike. Just know though that few moments on the lips can add more inches on the hips.

Eat wisely… especially late at night.

But if you do eat late, consider "*The Camel Diet*," and let that be what fuels you well into the late morning.

Sometimes it's about conscious balance.

To me, my *Camel Diet* is: eating enough to cross your metaphorical desert each day… instead of eating at regular, structured, and set times… especially if you don't know when your next meal might be.

That's why I try to get my work done before I allow myself to take time off to eat a meal. I make it the carrot at the end of a stick that I do reward myself with after doing a good job.

Sometimes we need those nuggets.

"*Food for fellowship*" is different than calories for sustenance.

So while a "*when in Rome*" attitude can be needed, be balanced.

The Religion-Obesity Connection

Recently, there was a TV report on a scientific paper published which followed teenagers into their adult years... half who went to church regularly... and half who were spiritual but not conventionally religious. The report told how those who thrive within the church and in religious life also stand a 50% greater chance of becoming obese.

That really raised my eyebrows. My reason for this? In church, food is one of the few "*safe*" addictions.

In other words, it's more socially acceptable to be addicted to food and fat than it is to reek of reefer or smell of alcohol and cigarettes. Unfortunately, I learned that the hard way too.

When I decided to join my church's praise group, I immediately noticed that I was the thinnest member of the band. They were mostly all relatively obese to some degree, and the leader also smoked cigarettes. Being that I did too, I enjoyed our smoke breaks... but noticed that over time, I was starting to gain a lot of weight while being in the band. Also, I developed an asthmatic wheeze during that stretch. It's almost as if the environment subconsciously encouraged me to not mind packing on a few pounds. As my priest noticed with a wink and a smile, "*You're ripening nicely Brian.*"

It was when we were performing a song with "*taste and see, taste and see... the goodness of the Lord*" in it that I realized I needed to make a change. Something about those lyrics made me look at those around me and wonder if taking some time away would help precipitate a change.

It did.

It was almost as if those you associate with often can be "*triggers*" towards the choices you make. Thus, if you want to make changes, a lot of times you have to go out and make new friends while disassociating from the old ones. While that may hurt, the important thing is that you're making such a change in your social circle to break the bad habits their social osmosis allows to seep into soul through the ritualistic acceptance they often can provide.

It's similar to going to a Weight Watchers meeting and then going a buffet… or like going to an Alcoholics Anonymous meeting and hitting the bar after.

The same principle applies.

And it drives me totally nuts when overly religious people who are obese vocally pray out loud for "*those poor alcoholics and drug addicts*" in church. Are they blind to see their own vices of gossip and overeating? Ever notice how a lot of priests become fat? If they can't have sex and aren't supposed to do drugs, what else is there for them to "*escape*"? Life is tough. We all tend to find a habit to help take the edge off a hard day.

We may be human… but we're still animals. And as animals, we still have habitual rituals we run to in order to escape the tough demands life tends to place on us.

That's one reason I totally agreed with the religion-obesity epidemic scientific story that I heard about on the news a year ago. Those who tend to have religion as one of their three primary habits only have two other habits turn to in tough times… and food, coffee, TV, telephone, and internet now tend to be the safest ones for them that seem to be tolerated.

Recently in attending a weekday morning mass, I decided to volunteer to help some of the church ladies prepare the weekend flyer. One of them has become so obese that she now needs one of those motorized scooters to get around and to go to church. So as we were chatting while preparing the flyers, she mentioned how the police stopped her in her scooter chair and told her she was impeding traffic while on her way to the library… which is less than a mile away from where she lives.

She pleaded, *"So what am I supposed to do now?"* I said, *"You can always walk."* She sounded shocked and exclaimed, *"I can't do that!"* I replied, *"You can; you just don't <u>think</u> you can."* She got very angry at that remark. All I was offering her was the truth. Hard work is exactly that – hard work. Yet deferred joys purchased through sacrifice are often the sweetest.

You can always walk.
You can always try harder.
You can always believe in yourself.

And the best thing about those concepts above?

They're all free. The best things in life always are.

Matter don't matter. The best things in life aren't things.

The thing is, I am a very spiritual person, and I tend to love *all* religions. Even though I was raised Catholic, I see each different religion as a different facet to the same diamond – God. He made us with so much potential to achieve elegant integrity… but He also instilled in us Free Will.

Sometimes those choices from our own free will lead us to poor directions and bad habits. So no matter how far down the wrong road you go, being willing to turn back.

Mother Teresa of Calcutta: *"While I might not have made a difference to everyone in the world, to those I helped, it meant the <u>whole</u> world."*

If you lose a few times, don't lose the lesson you learn.

<u>Why Do I Need Yet Another Addiction?</u>

Habit is replaced by habit… pure and simple.

If you give one up, you will pick up another in time.

The goal is to exchange all the bad ones for good ones.

Anything you intake into your 5 senses can be considered a drug. My feeling is that we each have 3 habits… making us all addicts of some sort. So the goal isn't to point fingers at people with other addictions… but to help each other become the best we can because we're all in it together.

Thus in my opinion, everyone is a drug addict.
Most of 'em just don't think that they are.
Most of them are in complete denial.
Habit is always replaced by habit.

If you have a bad habit and want to replace it with a good one, start hitting the gym more. It can become a habitual ritual that offers a healthy replacement for an addiction that can turn into a downward spiral. Replace a bad habit with a good one.

And I definitely feel that everyone has 3 primary addictions or habits that make up any given day. They are anything we do in excess to escape via the five sensory inputs we can receive. Some people debate me on that, but from what I've witnessed, it tends to be more true than false. In my opinion, virtual habits will sooner overshadow a lot of illegal drugs we've run to for years in order to escape. An example of this is my mom's craving for FarmVille and/or Facebook. Those can be considered two prime addictions for many these days.

People gotta get that virtual social media fix these days.
Can over a billion people be wrong? Frequently.

In my opinion, virtual addictions will soon overshadow all others. We'll recall how *"back in the day"* we just used to get high or drunk. We can all get misled about the latest bandwagon to jump on. In essence, a lot of those addictions, whatever they may be, just detour you from the focus necessary to achieve excellent and elegant integrity in more important aspects of life… such as diet, exercise, and creativity.

For example, a lot of labels like to mislead… they like to embellish so things sound healthier than they are… and it's funny that foods without labels (fresh fruits and vegetables) tend to be the healthiest. *"Broccoli doesn't brag,"* is a slogan I heard on Dr. Oz recently… but it's true… because it doesn't need to. Also notice that broccoli doesn't have a social media page for you to give a *"thumbs up"* or a *"like"* to… it just quietly goes about its business of being an excellent food source of vitamins and minerals. Quiet confidence often sells itself.

But like the saying goes, *"Peace sells, who's buying?"*

My political science teacher once asked our class, *"Is peace an interruption of war, or is war an interruption of peace?"*

Or as the Pink Floyd song says:
"Mother should I trust the government?

In the case of the FDA (Food and Drug Administration) the answer tends to be *yes*. They're often the ones who verify claims that may be bogus and order changes from those guilty of false advertising or misleading the consumer.

The same line of thought extends to a lot of food manufacturers who want you to become customers. As the movie *Scarface* reminds: *"Never underestimate the other guy's greed."*

That's one reason people and companies give away free samples. They want you to *"like"* it. They *want* to hook you.

When someone tries to give me something for free, my response tends to be: "*Why would I need yet another addiction?*"

Like a coke addict told me when I was trying to kick the habit: "*One hit is too many and a million is never enough.*" In other words, don't get the gorilla on your back to begin with. All it takes is one delightful experience for you to become a consistent customer and a constant consumer for life. That's where Nancy Reagan's "*Just Say No*" makes most sense… but if we consider everything we ingest via our 5 senses to be drugs, that slogan takes on a whole new meaning. Something to consider as you use those coupons that entice you to try a new product or accept a free sample at the store.

They want your business… period.

And they tend not to give you anymore free samples after you're hooked. Why would they? They already got what they wanted… an addict of their product… regardless of the nutritional claims their label may tout.

Today you may drink their wine.
Tomorrow you may be picking their grapes.

So remember that oatmeal is often better than no meal if your addiction starts hitting your pocketbook heavy like some can.

And if you want to give up a bad habit, start considering which one you'll want to take its place.

Habit is only replaced by another habit.

Be Good to Yourself at least Once Daily

One thing I have loved about going to church often during my life is that one of the gregarious nuns in my parish loves to tell me each time I hug her, *"Brian, be good to yourself today."* She always emphasizes the word **"good"** when she uses it too.

And while I've raised some issues with religion and church, the fact is, attending church frequently *has* helped me kick many bad addictions. Saying you want to change gives it power.

It was in the confessional that I began many bouts of abstinence. Yet that doesn't mean we still can't be good to ourselves daily.

In thinking about this book as I write it, I'm struck by how deadlines often get us to be our most productive when the moment is now. When it's appropriate, those all-nighters are often when our best work gets done. But when I'm in that zone, I realize that I often need and desire that nugget that keeps me coming back... that carrot at the end of the stick.

It's almost as if I provide little inch-pebble rewards for myself to keep the momentum flowing in order to make that deadline's milestone. That's a case where I'd be hard to dissuade you from bad diet decisions.

That's a case where crunch-time dictates the need to fuel yourself with whatever gets the job done on time, right, and with safe results for all. Again, it's a sense of a spoonful of sugar to get that medicine down... or to get that milestone achieved.

Like the Michael Keaton jokes in his *"Mr. Mom"* movie: *"Ah, 210, 220... whatever it takes"* in reference to being asked how he's going to rewire his house.

The whole point is to get back to work after you reward yourself with whatever is your appropriate nugget to entice you to do

your best before the deadline looms large. Or "*Get 'er done!*"
as Larry the Cable Guy reminds.

It's a case of being good to yourself… at least once a day.

That's because life is tough enough as it is… and taking the
edge off isn't always the bad thing that society can make it out
to be. If it gets you through a difficult day, can you rationalize it
away? That train of thought recently occurred when I met an
old high school friend for lunch with a beer in my hand. She
said, "*Boy, I wish I could do that… have a liquid lunch.*" I
responded, "*You can; you just don't think you can.*"

Just remember that if you do meet those milestones after
rewarding yourself, and decide to reward yourself again and
again with the cash windfall you may receive: *Big money can
bring bigger waistlines*.

Like Robin Williams said to some of his students in "*Dead
Poets Society*," "*Sucking the marrow out life doesn't mean
choking on the bone.*"

Life likes it when you sing and dance within the Music of the
Spheres that it provides, and it doesn't seem to mind a treat or
two to help you reach your goal. At least that's what I've
noticed. It often throws you a few Scoobie Snax as a reward.
When I realize such a special neat-to-eat cosmic-treat, I like to
say: "*That's as cool as the other side of the pillow.*"

So when in doubt, dance!
Be willing to sing badly.
Be good to yourself today.
If you don't, who will?

Success begets success… so act like you've been there before…
and realize that if you can't sing it, you can't play it.

Soda, Sugar, Sodium, Smoking, and Energy Drinks

Prior to writing this chapter, I was listening to Neil Young's song about a junkie – "_The Needle and the Damage Done._" In essence, its metaphor can be applied to us all in one area of addiction (or habitual ritual) or another. We all have a fatal flaw, and is it too late to turn back now?

One of my friends thinks so. He was diagnosed with cancer recently, and he was absolutely convinced it was from the chemicals in diet soda. His complete recovery after surgery caused me a complete reassessment of how I was living. Facing mortality, yours or a close friend's, tends to do that. I think Steve Jobs' death did that for a lot of us too. Such a passing causes us to actively consider how we can do things better now... sooner, rather than later. Do it now before it's too late, because if you have to go under the knife to remove it, you obviously didn't act soon enough.

An ounce of prevention is worth a pound of cure, right? So let's take a look at the labels of soup. I now call it _liquid sodium_.

Teach yourself to taste sodium. But first, be aware of it.

Thus, a dry roasted almond is worse than a raw one.

Wean yourself off so your taste becomes sharpened.

Conscious awareness through touch, taste, and feel is crucial.

Sugary drinks and energy drinks produce an empty crash. Be aware of it. Can you gain energy another way? If you cut one 20-ounce sugary soda or energy drink from your diet every day of the year, you'll save over 80,000 calories during that year that you don't have to diet or exercise off. It's often all about that ratio of nutrients to calories.

So the moral of the story is: Don't drink your fruits and vegetables... eat them. They're a lot healthier where you're actually eating them as the Earth provides. The more mankind cleaves something natural; the more side-effects there tend to be that we humans have to deal with.

Like a girlfriend of mine said, "*A glass of wine is fine... just don't drink the whole bottle.*" The same applies with coffee and dark chocolate. Both contain incredible anti-oxidants, but too much of any one thing is bad. Be aware of your inner fulcrum.

One thing I definitely recommend is going on mini-fasts where you completely abstain from a habit you tend to think you can't do without. For example, I'm known to my close friends as being somewhat of a Diet Pepsi junkie. I love getting my cold caffeine fix of fizz and carbonation. I was really surprised though of being able to taste the chemicals in diet soda after two weeks away without it whatsoever. I did this after reading a report on Yahoo about the effects of even one can of diet cola soda a day. It said that even one simple bottle of diet cola a day can raise blood pressure long-term.

To me, it's all because artificial sweeteners tend to trick your brain. Also, all those chemicals with names I can't even try to pronounce in a can of diet soda cause me to believe that, as much as I love them, I can do better.

The trick becomes acting on such knowledge.
Easier said than done.

One way I made it through two weeks without diet soda was to invest in lots and lots of sparkling water... because even diet tonic water has artificial sweeteners, and club soda has a lot more sodium than you'd expect.

Like I've mentioned before; habit is only replaced by habit.

If I'm not willing to give up carbonation, where can I get my bubbles elsewhere? Sparkling water? Beer? Ahem...

It's as if we're damned if we do and damned if we don't. Where's the fine line between enjoyment and good health?

When diet and exercise aren't enough though, check your sodium… as a bodybuilder reminded, *"It makes a difference when dieting down for a competition to watch your salt and fluids days prior to the contest."*

It tends to be a hidden culprit that many of us don't seem to consider. Also, from the reports I've seen and read, our culture overdoses on sodium constantly.

Hydration – This is such a crucial cure that most ignore.

There's a huge importance in drinking water when it comes to weight loss… drink a few glasses of H2O before meals… it fills you up and helps you eat less calories when the food arrives. Moreover, it helps detoxify your body and rid your system of pollutants quickly. If you do, consider Kegels too.

Once you start going to the bathroom a lot, Kegels strengthen those important bladder control muscles that can be an issue later in life.

Back when I first started watching my weight, I subscribed to the *Eat to Win* approach of filling your body with complex carbs in order to achieve excellence in endurance athletics. Since I played competitive racquetball, that idea really worked for me. I had the fuel to make it through a weekend of racquetball tournament matches because I ate smart prior to my matches. Then came *The Zone Diet* and Balance Bars that gave a more well-rounded dieting approach. Then I liked *The Atkins Diet* because of its lean protein advice that helped my muscles grow at the gym. After that, I heard about the 90/10 food philosophy… which allows for 10% luscious indulgence in fun foods. Give wiggle room for the jiggle in the middle.

All in all, each one has its time and place. Each is appropriate to the goals you're trying to achieve. Just remember that when it comes to diet, we all tend to fall off the wagon at one time or another. The goal becomes to enjoy those mini-diet-vacations, and then get back to work eating right after you've given yourself the rewards you crave.

So reward yourself once you give up a bad addiction. If you quit smoking, do the math on an average of about 10 packs a week… which in Michigan at about $7/pack adds up to a savings of approximately $300 a month… or over $3000 saved a year. Now if you go to Manhattan in NYC where the cost is over $10 per pack, the bang for your buck goes up in terms of what you're saving by giving up something you want… but don't need. The interesting conundrum with rewarding yourself after a goal is reached is that it may create a trending slide or fall from grace. You reach a peak and then reward yourself and start slacking off a bit. It happens to us all. The point is to be consciously aware of it and to minimize such slides when they arrive… because life is always a sinusoidal ebb and flow.

A metaphor to consider when making such rewards for yourself and reaching your goals is to think about the children's game "*Chutes & Ladders.*" Just like I often see the world as huge versions of Bill Murray's movie "*Groundhog Day*" and the game of "*Chutes & Ladders*" where we consciously have to learn our lessons in order to continue climbing to the top and make it to the next day… while avoiding the nasty slides along the way that life likes to throw at us to see which way we wiggle, jiggle, and decide.

Remember: "*Any smart man can get himself out of a jam, but it's the intelligent man who avoids the problem all together.*"

One way I gave up some bad habits was to cut my hair. It helped me to see a new man in the mirror. So while cutting my long hair may seem drastic, I was willing to do whatever it took to let go of many bad habits. I had to face myself in the mirror and remind myself why my hair was short now.

For example, when I used to smoke a lot, I dated a beautiful woman who smoked too. As we were coming home, I told her I wanted to stop at the store because I needed a pack of cigarettes. She said, "*No. You don't _need_ a pack of cigarettes; you _want_ a pack of cigarettes.*" That kind of conscious realization helped.

A similar line of thought is to *want* to diet... rather than feeling that you *have* to diet. It's a paradigm shift that introduces new ways of thinking but adapting such thoughts tend to take time... especially over a lifetime.

It's one thing to say it. It's another thing entirely to do it.

So only talk the talk if you intend on walking the walk.

A patent attorney told me in regards to a patent idea: "*First, go out and make it. Build a working prototype. Because when it gets right down to law, you can't really patent or copyright an idea... but you can patent or copyright the execution of an idea.*" Then he said, "*For example, one great idea is to make a pill that you put in water so it turns to gasoline. Make that pill, and you'll make a fortune.*"

In other avenues, in recently speaking with a spinning instructor about this "*Dessert First Diet,*" she asked me why she feels so bad about eating ice cream... after she eats it. My response concluded that it's more of a psychosomatic symptom. In other words, she knows how long it will take to burn off the calories she just ate because she makes her living and pays her bills because of exercise and staying in shape. Thus, even though she loves its taste, she stresses over the way it will make her look and how much work needs to be done... instead of savoring the reward she's providing to her soul.

For example, here near Detroit, there is literally a Hell, Michigan that I drove to on a 100 degree day. The people there usually like to joke about how it's hot as hell there, but since their air conditioning wasn't working, their humor wasn't humoring them. However, with it being "*99 in the Shade*" (a Bon Jovi song I listened to on that drive to Hell and back), the taste of that ice cream waffle cone was one of my best delicacies in recent memory… simply because it was an earned reward… deferred joys purchased through sacrifice are often the sweetest. That day, that ice cream at 2pm, on an empty stomach, in triple digit temperatures, with no air conditioning, was *The Best!*

The whole point to remember is that retraining ourselves to live differently takes time and practice. It takes making mistakes to realize how we made them… so we don't repeat them again.

And while I've used my overweight mother as an example in this book often, the fact is that this book wouldn't exist without her and her unconditional love and support for my vision of becoming a successful author… even after almost everyone else told me I was crazy… and that I should go back to my old life as a successful engineer. In other words, sometimes it requires a lot of growing pains to metamorphosize and transform into someone new… someone better… someone you love when you look in the mirror. Just don't give up. Change is never easy.

Just be compassionate to those at least trying to try.
Cheerlead them and offer encouragement.
They may be your next visionary.

You never know if your college drop-out or that homeless bum will become our next Einstein or our next Basquiat. And as Jean-Michel Basquiat is quoted as saying, "*Many young kings get their heads cut off.*" If you've seen the movie "*The Man Who Would Be King,*" you know exactly what I mean.

Coda and Conclusions - The Dessert First Diet

Wow...

What a nice journey it's been sharing all this info with you!

I definitely have grown in the process of jotting it all down, transcribing all those notes to my manuscript, editing them, and then elaborating on each point to share with you.

I truly hope that these nuggets of common sense have helped. That's really what it's all about... becoming better people. If I knew then what I know now, would I do it the same?

You bet, _but I certainly wouldn't want to repeat it._ (haha!)

So if there's one nugget I really think you should live by after reading all this, it'd be to not live your life asking _"what if?"_ because life is too short to be second-guessing yourself with woulda's, shoulda's, and coulda's.

In other words, live a life without regret.

To do that takes making active choices – consistently. If you were to die today, would your soul be at peace? You can't build a reputation on what you are going to do.

If not, then _"Now!"_ is the time to make a change... not tomorrow, not later... because if you live your life saying _"Tomorrow,"_ you'll never get a chance to truly enjoy any Yesterdays. If you always travel the Streets of By-and-By, you _will_ eventually arrive at the House of Never.

That last paragraph's wisdom was shared with me recently by one of my old math professors in undergrad after she spent some time recovering from a serious illness that had her come face-to-face with her own mortality.

With that said, let's wrap this puppy up with some more nuggets of wisdom with which you can march on into the sunset with your head held high.

First, when I recently had my body-mass-index (BMI) measure by a gym trainer who had lost over 60 pounds, her philosophy was that weight loss is 80% diet, 10% exercise, and 10% genetics… personally, I disagree with that ratio (thinking exercise should be a greater percentage and diet a slightly lower percentage), but her "*before*" and "*after*" photos speak volumes… so who am I to argue with the philosophy that worked for her… thus, be willing to modify your ratios.

It's all about what works for you.
It's all about being sustainable.
It's all about being healthier.

One thing that I like about this food philosophy is that it enabled me to be "*in the zone*" more often and on a more consistent basis with endurance.

There are those shining moments of being "*in the zone*" – when you're glad to be alive. And that's a lot of what this book is all about. Learning what it takes a lot of practice to develop the muscle memory to make wise choices out in the world on-the-fly and without a lot of thought.

It's as if you train your body to act naturally so everything just flows when the money is on the line. It's a *drive for show, putt for dough* mentality. In other words, our diets can often be penny-wise and pound-foolish… both literally and figuratively. So can our training regimens. Wise wins. Consider the tale of the Tortoise and the Hare… sometimes slow wins too.

As a priest reminded me when I was homeless in 1999, "*God's wisdom is slow learning so the roots grow strong and deep.*" While it wasn't what I wanted to hear while sleeping out on the beach next to the sea, he was right.

And now that those days are over, I wouldn't trade those tough times for the world. That doesn't mean that I want to repeat them though either; trust me.

Right before I left my engineering job in LA back in 1995, a fellow engineer and I were having breakfast in Brentwood, a ritzy part of LA where I lived for 9 months. After eating my meal and pushing my plate away that still had food on it, he noticed and said the following: *"That's actually a lesson some young princes are taught... to push the plate away even if there's food still left on it. You and I, we were raised in the Midwest where it was always a rule to clean your plate."*

What my friend taught me was a conscious self-control.

Actively acknowledge that we don't need to eat it all.

It's that *"drive for show, putt for dough"* thing again.

Act like you've been there before. Quiet confidence.

Since *"Wise Wins"* for me, here's some more wisdom my racquetball coaches shared with me when I was playing tournaments, earning sponsorships, and winning: *"Don't play the weekend warrior if you want to get better... get beat by the best instead... and sooner or later, they won't be beating you because you'll have taken your game up a notch or two. If all you do is go slummin' you'll always be in the slums."*

One also encouraged over a few amber ales: *"The score is merely a time-keeping device. It simply tells you when to go on the court and when to come off it. What matters is that you truly love the game you play."*

In trying to locate him in Michigan's upper peninsula a few months ago, I learned by looking in the Yellow Pages that his address was on *"1234 Harley Davidson Drive,"* and in Mapquesting it, realized that he'd given a bogus address that was really yet another piece of Zen. I finally got the joke.

When the pupil is ready, a master will appear.

The master always continues to teach.

It's whether we're willing to listen.

Did you know that a chronic lack of rest can actually make you sick? That's another concept I can across during the writing of this book that I thought I should share. Make sure you get your sleep. While there are times we must burn the midnight oil, we *do* need our downtimes to recuperate.

As physics suggests: *a body at rest tends to stay at rest, and a body in motion tends to stay in motion.*

If we're always at One, what do you do to get back to Zero?

My term for such reverse-psychology is "*Perspectives of Scale*" where we see things from a different perspective… street level versus an airplane POV. If every side of you can agree on the finished product, and from all angles it seems correct, chances are that you have completed your task correctly.

First on, last off when it comes to weight gain and weight loss.

That's a concept I read about in Muscle & Fitness back in 1986 when I was a freshman in college. It refers to "*stack*" thinking that Hewlett-Packard calculators are famous for… but it also refers to our bodies and how they tend to store fat. Where you put it on first will be where it comes off last as you melt away the fat with dieting and exercise.

For a man, you'll tend to loose those love handles last. For a woman, those moments on the lips first tend to show up in your legs and hips.

It's all about masculine and feminine genetics.
Where the sexes tend to store their fat.

First on, last off… it's a fact.

When I first lost a lot of weight over this past year using this *Dessert First Diet* approach, one way I noticed it was when I had to cinch my baseball cap up a notch. I joked about it by saying, "*Wow, what a fat head I had!*"

The fact is: we accumulate fat *all over*.

The fact that I had to cinch my hat showed that.

There's always a reason for the season… when you're on top of the world, there's nowhere to go but down. When you're at rock bottom, there's no where to go but up. The people you mistreat on the way up may be the ones you meet on the way down. Balance and karma do exist. Act wisely.

Concede you're going to lose a few battles of the muffin-top bulge. What matters is that you win the lifelong weight loss war... and it *is* a war that we often become POW's from… because food *can* hold us hostage.

Remember: Life is a marathon not a sprint.

Think about why a light bulb eventually fails. Really, it's from the cycling of going from to "*off*" and "*on*" too many times. If it were to always stay on, it'd tend to last a lot longer. That's simply because the up and down states require lots of warm-ups and cool-downs that push it into the red.

Being "*in the red*" is when mistakes and mishaps tend to occur most. Don't push yourself too far, too fast. Slow down so the roots grow strong and deep.

A lot of people *can* get back in shape… they just don't *think* they can. One way to do so is to stick around similar people with like-minded motivations. That's one reason I like being at the gym. It's an environment conducive to positive change and good amounts of growth in the right way. While there are always those who tend to take short-cuts, the fact remains that many are there doing it the old fashioned way – earning it with lots of hard work.

Studies have shown that attitude, determination, and intensity do factor into getting better scores on IQ tests. Consider that when you diet or train.

While you can't measure hope, morality, belief, attitude, and confidence, when you just naturally exude these qualities, people can tell. They speak for themselves.

That's why there's always a reason for the season. It's also one reason that I like living in my home town of Detroit, Michigan. Here, you definitely experience all four seasons, and they make for a robust sense of personality. Be a Man of All Seasons.

After a long, cold wintertime…
The euphoria of spring? Earned.
The same with your body. Earn it.

It's only by slugging through a long and tough winter that spring's sense of new growth really means *more* for those who *endure* the snow and cold.

The best things in life are worth enduring to earn.

Your body is a seasonal thing which *needs* its earned endurance. Also worth enduring is the process which teaches you to *learn how to learn.*

One thing one of my graduate school advisors told me when I was considering getting my doctoral degree was that his PhD taught him that he can teach himself whatever he sets his mind on. Do you feel that way too?

Teach by example. Go out and be a Passion Hero… at times, use words. Write your own book of life. How many chapters do you want it to be? Also, are you willing to change your story if you're not satisfied?

Wisdom with hindsight... begin to see data trends over time.

Cravings are a fact of life. We covet what we see every day.

With this being the case, don't be jealous of others if they've done well. Instead of pointing fingers, become the change you want to see in the world. If you do, the results will eventually manifest themselves in such an elegant way that you'll be **Glad** you made the changes... because you *wanted* to.

Think about going a gym or health club because the fact of surrounding yourself with people who create a common collective of intensity to make a positive change in themselves seeps into your soul like a good osmosis.

While everyone can go on a specific diet and lose a lot of weight fast, the goal of the *Dessert First Diet* is more about feeding your soul with what it truly craves while making smart choices afterwards for bodily balance.

It's about a lifetime of living sustainably with a healthy attitude. If your mind isn't in it, it really doesn't matter how hard you try.

Love is passion and when you do something you love, it shows... so make something that represents "*the Ideal.*" Confidence and hard work do pay off, and the consistency of vision and values is worth being real and true.

Live an active life, not a passive one. Think smart.

Park further away for the additional benefits of walking.

Do so much more with less. Just the gist. Less is more.

After learning a lot of these lessons from my racquetball coach back in the day, he opened up his palm up to me and said with a smile: "*You may take the pebble Grasshopper.*" It *does* take a character to have Character.

Believe in yourself. Know that you can do it.

Because if you don't believe in yourself, who will?

Leadership is to go where there is no path and leaving a trail.

I hope that the trail you leave will be one of inspiration, transformation, and change that people will want to follow. Leaders do that. They are the ones who realize you all may be in the wrong forest (lesson: see the forest through the trees), while the managers are the ones who are happy to be making progress in the one they're in… regardless of if it's wrong.

Another concept to consider: When you go to the store, do you read labels, or do you expect everything to be spoon-fed for you? Are you actively conscious of what you're ingesting? If not, start paying more attention. You <u>can</u> always start Today.

Always ask yourself about new diet fads: "*Is it sustainable?*"

You don't want to hop on a bandwagon that happens to be heading off a cliff. Consider the common sense of whether it sounds too good to be true.

If it sounds too good to be true, it usually is. You can't get something from nothing. As my mom likes to say, "*The dirt always comes out in the wash.*" Or "*Good from far, but far from good,*" as my racquetball coach would say.

It's the space inside that gives any bowl its value… choose wisely what you fill it with. That's where that empty space becomes premium. Sometimes I guess, you just have to dump out the contents and to refill it again.

In poker, they say that it's not how many hands you play… but the quality of choices you make in the hands you *do* play.

The Game of Life is one meant to be played. It's not one you want to be caught sitting on the sidelines watching. Don't talk about being great unless you can actually go out and be Great... 24-7. Walk that walk... and *when* you do (not *if*), it *may* sound cocky to others, but to you it will just be *Truth*.

Food for thought...

Remember, this is not a diet.
It's *a new food philosophy*.

Choose smarter, not harder.
Dessert First Diet.

Cure those cravings before they blossom into big binges.

I wish you the best always and blessings for wise choices and healthy decisions. Believe that you can make the positive changes in your life that produce a silent smile.

If you think you can't... you're right.
If you believe you can... you're right.
Is your glass half empty or is it half full.

You *are* that little train that could.
You *can* make the necessary changes.

Thank you for reading my book:

"Dessert First Diet"

I truly hope it helps you precipitate a change for the better. But I also pray that it enables you to enact a healthy attitude to food.

All the very best,
Brian Shell

Books by the Author – Brian Shell

Detour
Gratitude Miles
From Student to Engineer
Crossing through Career Crossroads
Single Mom Soul – Spring
Single Mom Soul – Summer
Single Mom Soul – Autumn
Single Mom Soul – Winter
All Men Are Dogs
Cubicle Cardio
The Chip
Love Poems
Mind Games
Here & There
Teenage Jesus
Facebook Diaries
Dessert First Diet
Start My Heart Art
American Romance
Up from the Snakepit
A Prodigal Son Returns
Single Mom Daily Devotions
Texas Hold'em Tournament Tactics
Oprah and I – My Own A-Ha Moment
Shastras – Received Wisdom about *Right* Conduct
Pre-Celebrity Jesus – The Man before the Messiah
Attack of the Electronic Dust Bunnies
A Juxtaposition of Idiosyncrasies
The Sexuality of Synergy
Making a Masterpiece
Distortions

www.ingramcontent.com/pod-product-compliance
Lightning Source LLC
Chambersburg PA
CBHW070402290526
45790CB00004B/1598